Running Until You Are 100

By
Terence McCarthy

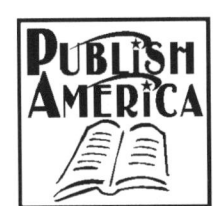

PublishAmerica
Baltimore

© 2009 by Terence McCarthy.
All rights reserved. No part of this book may be reproduced, stored in a retrieval system or transmitted in any form or by any means without the prior written permission of the publishers, except by a reviewer who may quote brief passages in a review to be printed in a newspaper, magazine or journal.

First printing

This publication contains the opinions and ideas of its author. Author intends to offer information of a general nature. Neither the author nor the publisher are engaged in rendering medical, health or any other kind of personal professional services to the reader. The reader should consult his or her own physician before relying on any information set forth in or implied from this publication. Any reliance on the information herein is at the reader's own discretion.

The author and publisher specifically disclaim all responsibility for any liability, loss, or right, personal or otherwise, which is incurred as a consequence, directly or indirectly, of the use and application of any contents of this book. They further make no representations or warranties with respect to the accuracy or completeness of the contents of this work and specifically disclaim all warranties including without limitation any implied warranty of fitness for a particular purpose. Any recommendations are made without any guarantee on the part of the author or the publisher.

PublishAmerica has allowed this work to remain exactly as the author intended, verbatim, without editorial input.

ISBN: 978-1-4489-2420-2 (softcover)
ISBN: 978-1-4489-9373-4 (hardcover)
PUBLISHED BY PUBLISHAMERICA, LLLP
www.publishamerica.com
Baltimore

Printed in the United States of America

Running Until You Are 100

Foreword

The author of this article has spent over 37 years as an active runner. In his mid-seventies he is still competitive. Last year he competed in 29 road races and was first in his age group (70-74 years) in 23 of those contests.

Over the years he has amassed a great deal of data in experience and research. Many different sources are used in compiling the information in this guide from medical journals, newspaper health items and several running publications. His personal experience is also a major factor.

The purpose of this comprehensive guide is to suggest a disciplined and pro-active program for you to consider if you are seriously interested in running until you reach 100 years of age. It is vital that you adopt a program that fits your circumstances and physical condition.

The overriding rationale for you to take a dynamic role in this process is the following assumption: approximately seventy percent of how long we can be active running enthusiasts depends on the choices we make. The other 30%—our genes—is beyond our control.

Looking Forward to Century-Old Runners

In the 1980's, most organized running races had age groups that topped out at 40 years and over. In the early 1990's, the majority of the races recognized the oldest age group as 50 and over. After 1995 more events included the 60 and over age group. After the year 2000, the top age group moved closer to 70 and over with some establishing the top age group award at 80-99. The trend to more older and aged runners has truly been astounding.

When I started running in earnest in 1971, I was stationed at the Pentagon and was informed that I had orders to go to parachute training (jump school) at Fort Benning, Georgia. At that time there were just a few active runners over 50 years of age. By the year 2015, there will be a significant number of runners in their 90's. Extending this "old geezer" hyperactivity to the year 2025, we can reasonably expect to see numerous 100 year olds still running (not very fast) road races!!!

Currently (the year is 2009) I am in my mid-seventies and expect to be one of those running competitively when I reach 100 years of age. Granted, the number of active runners will diminish in the later years due to injuries, disabilities and death. However, there is reason to believe that more runners will be able to remain active longer IF they adopt a disciplined and effectively tailored program to fit his (her) own physiological and environmental needs.

The purpose of this article is to recommend guidelines for runners 55 and over which, if followed and pragmatically implemented, will assist more runners to successfully reach the century age plateau in their running careers. The most important thing to bear in mind is that the application of these suggested guidelines must be tailored to fit the individual's circumstances and needs. Some of these may not work for you.

Section 1: Training Regimen

As we get older, the body and its components—especially, the joints and muscles—need diversity, replenishment and rest. A typical weekly training regimen needs to be designed to provide the basics such as:

Sunday: Day of rest. (This assumes that Saturday was a race day or a hard workout.)

PURPOSE: Prolong your running career.

Monday: Long Run Day. Plan on running a distance 1 mile longer than your next scheduled race. (Shut the run down at the 60 minute point.)

PURPOSE: Develop and maintain stamina.

Tuesday: Cross Training Exercise Day. Consider 30 minutes of swimming or cycling. I prefer swimming because of the benefit to your back and muscular structure.

PURPOSE: Provide alternative exercise to your running and prolong joint life.

Wednesday: Interval Training. Recommend 4 to 5 repetitions of ¼ mile walking and ¼ mile running. Conduct the ¼ mile run at a 1 to 1 ½ mile pace faster than your race pace. The treadmill is ideal for this activity.

NOTE: I have selected the ¼ mile segment which allows you to maximize the speed workout. I avoid sprints because they are too stressful on older joints and muscles.

PURPOSE: Maintain race pace.

Thursday: Day of rest.

PURPOSE: Prolong your running career.

Friday: (Assuming this is the day prior to race day) Do two repetitions of interval training.

PURPOSE: Acclimate body to faster race pace reflex. Prevent your race times from declining.

Saturday: Race day or hard work out similar to race experience.

PURPOSE: Maintain competitive status.

COMMENTARY: The typical training/race week needs to conserve your energy and keep your joints from a daily pounding exposure. Workouts and/or races of more than 60 minutes must be avoided. Back-to-back running days must be avoided. Two days of rest are mandatory so that the body can replenish itself from the exercise impacts. Thirty minute walks on your day of rest are okay if you feel up to doing it.

Concerning the restriction of hard workouts and running to sixty minutes, this statement is attributed to Dr. Cooper of the Cooper Clinic in Dallas, Texas. He said: "When you run up to sixty minutes, you are running for your health. When you run for more than sixty minutes, you are running for your ego."

This regimen is designed to support your running career into your 80's, 90's and even into your 100's.

Section 2: Cross Training

In order to prolong your running career, it is absolutely essential that you avoid back-to-back running days. Otherwise, you can expect serious erosion of joint proficiency over the long term. Repetitive day-to-day running (even of varying intensity) only increases the cumulative pounding and stress impact on your joints. The key point here is that repetitive day-to-day running over the age of 55 does not allow the joints to be replenished. This can only occur through rest and cross training.

Cross training allows the joints to work in a different physiological manner which enables the joints to recover from the hard-pounding running experience and to develop greater joint strength. There are several cross training activities that you can pursue. The two types of cross training recommended are: swimming and cycling. Thirty minute workouts are prescribed once or twice a week.

I prefer swimming because my sports therapist recommends crawl swimming as being much more beneficial to the muscular structure and especially in enhancing the pliability and loosening of the back muscles.

Cross training saved my knees from "going south" when I was 57 years old. Recommend you read Section 10: EXPERIENCE AND LESSONS LEARNED for more on this subject.

Section 3: Strength Training

As you go beyond your 55th year, running by itself becomes insufficient to maintain the optimum capabilities of your upper and lower body muscles. Muscle tissue, bone density and strength all diminish over the years. Sarcopenia—the gradual decrease in muscle tissue—actually begins at age 30. Tracking this loss of muscle mass, one can expect to lose about 25% of muscle mass and strength by age 70 and another 25% by age 90. The weakening of either the upper or lower group of body muscles can result in declining running performance achievement levels. My experience in Section 10 underscores specific examples of problems that can arise in this area.

Strength or weight resistance training is the most effective way to offset the physiological effects of aging. Without an established weight resistance program, the chances for running past 90 appear almost non-existent. Studies of older adults participating in strength training have shown that the decline in strength and muscle tissue mass can be recouped.

Resistance can be supplied by your body weight, free weights, elasticized bands or specialized machines. Weight resistance workouts are recommended at least two times a week. The length should last 10 to 15 minutes per workout. Always allow a minimum interval of 48 hours between workouts. You should develop at least three specific workouts for the upper and lower body muscles. Get advice from a trainer which sets will be most beneficial to your situation. In the use of specialized machines and weights, I strongly recommend: adduction—strengthens the inner thigh muscles, rowing, leg & ankle press, arm curl and bar bell press.

Strength training routines consist of lifting and lowering a weight 10 to 15 times or repetitions (reps); this constitutes one set. The complete workout will include one to two sets of 6 to 12 exercises. In doing each workout, choose the weight that allows you to do 10 to 15 reps. The last two reps should be difficult. If you can't lift the weight at least ten times, use a lighter weight. Once you can perform the reps with ease and without tiring the muscle, increase the amount of weight. Resting for a minute between sets will maximize strength gains. During the workout breathe out as you lift, and inhale as you lower weights. Never hold your breath. Lift weights to a three-second count. Pause for one second. Lower weights to a three second count. Always do a 5 to 10 minute warm up before each workout and cool down afterward. Remember the aim in this type of training is to always reach muscle fatigue at the end of each set.

Strength training gradually replaces fat with muscle. This results in big health dividends that will help to fight high blood pressure, heart disease, gall bladder disease, arthritis, diabetes and certain cancers.

Another training regimen is called power training. The basic procedure is to use weighted vests as you perform thrusts and other activities such as climbing stairs, walking and slow jogging. A small study in the *Journal of the American Geriatrics Society* in 2002 concluded that workouts using weighted vests improved power significantly in older adults.

Section 4: Periodic Maintenance

As you get older, the muscles in the calves, hamstrings, quadriceps and glutes accumulate tightness, sometimes, cramps over several months time. Most runners—even those who do stretching to the maximum—are unaware of this changing muscular condition. My first tip off that there is a problem, occurs when I stretch out my legs in bed at night and experience a temporary muscle spasm. Younger runners seem to recover more effectively and rarely experience this phenomenon.

The solution is a preventative process called "periodic maintenance". It is recommended that you visit a certified sports massage therapist every three or four months for a maintenance message. Normally, a thirty minute visit is sufficient to loosen up the calves, quadriceps, hamstrings and glutes. You will probably be amazed to discover how tight your muscles have become. It is strictly a product of aging.

It is important for you to establish your own frequency for your periodic maintenance visits. Some may find that every two months works better or perhaps every four months.

Section 5: Race Day Regimen

So much has been written on this subject that I will stress only the basics.

Hydration should start the night before and stop an hour and a half prior to race time. Five to ten minutes before the race begins, drink about five to six ounces of an energy drink.

Solid food should be ingested no later than two hours before race time so that the digestive process will have sufficient time to be completed.

Complete your stretching about 5 to 10 minutes before the race start. Spend a good 5 to 10 minutes in the stretching routine. For an effective technique, consult a personal trainer who can assist you in tailoring the right stretching package.

Warm up just prior to the race start is a real must. However, since your energy fuel tank is limited, keep this activity to a bare minimum. Walking or jogging in place will help to raise your heart rate to more desirable levels.

By doing intervals prior to race day, you should be able to establish a comfortable and somewhat competitive race pace.

When going up hills, maintain your race pace and shorten your stride. When running down hills, maintain your race pace and lengthen your stride. Running short steps going down hill puts undue strain on the quadriceps and the hamstrings. Sprinting down hills can cause you to over-strain your heart without any awareness. Avoid excessive down hill speeds. Psychologically, when running up hills, try not to look all the way up the hill. This can be demoralizing. Keep your head down and tell yourself that "this hill is nothing" and "I can do it". Since you normally don't have to worry about oncoming traffic, there is no real reason to look up a hill!!!

Take advantage of each water distribution point. On hot days take an extra cup of water and douse your head and face. You will notice an instant refreshment from this which will mentally "jump-start" your running pace.

About a mile to a mile and a half before the finish line you will want to raise your pace up a notch. The technique to consider is mentally force your foot to stretch out frontally, raise your knee and let your foot naturally hit the running surface. The use of this technique for a short distance seems to work without causing any undue stress or pain.

After the race, make sure you have an energy drink or take some sort of athletic performance supplement. Personally, for hard runs and races, I take a vitamin supplement which is called "Overdrive". It is primarily available through alternative medicine clinics and Nu Skin distributors. "Overdrive" supports optimal athletic performance and assists in post-exercise recovery. For normal body weight and exercise duration of 30 minutes to 1 hour, the recommended dosage is one tablet one hour prior to the exercise event and one tablet one hour after the exercise.

Another serious post race/hard workout consideration is massage therapy. Muscles produce lactic acid during intensive workouts. The more intense the workout, the more lactic acid is produced. The greater the accumulation of lactic acid, the more fatigued and painful the muscles become. Lactic acid will dissipate on its own. As you get into your 50's and older, this process works much more slowly. However, one way to offset the "lactic acid buildup" is by enhancing blood circulation through massage therapy. This therapy not only gets rid of lactic acid more quickly, but, helps to relieve muscle cramps and spasms. In addition, massage therapy promotes the release of endorphins, a natural sedative that alleviates pain and produces a general sense of well being. Experience has clearly proven that massage therapy is more beneficial as athletes get past their 55th birthday. Personally, I have found that a jacuzzi with strong jets and a water temperature of around 103 degrees also helps to dissipate lactic acid buildup by enhancing blood circulation. In addition, the endorphin release seems to be a pleasant benefit as well.

Post-race hydration is also vital. Remember that as you get older, the natural thirst stimulus declines. You need to establish a set routine of water intake after a hard workout or a race. Don't rely on your feeling thirsty to determine your liquid intake. A good indicator of your satisfactory hydration status is to check the color of your urine. Urine that is dark colored and smelly suggests you need to drink more fluids. If you are well hydrated, you will eliminate a light-colored urine every two to four hours.

Section 6: Running Shoes

When it comes to running and prolonging your running years, the most important running equipment is your shoes. Selecting the "right" shoes is vital to preventing physical problems and even disabilities.

Patronize a running store which personally fits the shoes and analyzes your running technique in any prospective shoes that you are considering. Always bring your most recently used running shoes into the store so that they can be evaluated as to wear patterns. This will be a great help in determining the type of replacement shoe that is needed to correct stability or motion deficiencies. Doing a practice run in the replacement shoes—preferably on a tread mill—will present you the best opportunity to evaluate and acquire the "right" shoes. This selection process will provide big dividends for you in extending your longevity in running over the coming years.

Replace your running shoes after 500 miles of use at a minimum. If you don't keep track of your running miles and are active on a weekly basis, consider replacing your running shoes every 8 to 10 months.

Even though price is important, don't consider for a moment going on your own to a sports equipment store and purchasing running shoes which are on sale. This is not the time to save money and ruin your running career.

Section 7: Running Surfaces

Another key factor in running until you are 100 years old, is the type of surface you consistently run on. Your joints—especially the knees and hip joints—are very sensitive to the pounding impact of hard surfaces and are more inclined to look more kindly at softer, pliable surfaces.

A given is that you don't have a say in the running surfaces that race events use. However, you do have the prerogative to select the type of running surface on which you do your training runs. What type of surface should you consider and what type of running surface should you avoid?

First, let's look at surfaces that you should avoid. Never—I say NEVER—run on concrete, astro-turf, brick or flagstone surfaces. These surfaces provide the most intense and damaging pressures on your joints and muscle structure. Black tar pavement is not as severe but still should be avoided.

Second, the recommended running surfaces are: treadmills, wood chip trails and dirt/gravel trails Obviously, treadmills afford you the best running environment. Here, you can control the race pace and the incline. The pliability of the surface provides the lowest joint impact pressures. The next best surface is wood chip trails. The softness and pliability of this surface is very kind to your joints. The last surface in this recommended category is dirt/gravel trails. This type of surface is relatively easy to find. I have been running on horse trails for the past 26 years and believe that this type of surface has helped immeasurably to keep my joints from developing serious problems.

Section 8: Diet

Eating a performance-enhancing diet isn't easy. For many runners, nutrition is a huge missing link. Always eat breakfast. This is the most important meal of the day. Within three hours of getting up, have a full snack on good energy food like a whole grain cereal plus milk and fruit—an ideal carb-protein combination.

Carbohydrates are essential to your energy diet and help to resupply energy to your muscles. Be sure to include the "good carbs" in your diet such as pasta, potatoes, whole wheat bread and bagels. Muscles store carbs as glycogen. Glycogen depletion is associated with fatigue. Don't forget to include protein which is an important part of the sports diet and is needed for recovery from hard workouts. Remember that carbs are the foundation of the recovery meal and protein in smaller portions should always accompany carbs.

Don't get hooked on energy bars. Bananas, yogurt, fig newtons and granola bars are just as good and offer a great fuel source at prices that are more affordable.

Hydrating yourself is a must. Dehydration slows you down. Plan to drink extra fluids before you exercise. The kidneys require up to 90 minutes to process fluids. Make the appropriate time allowances before a race or an intense workout. Gatorade and other sports drinks are good for runners during extended exercise and should not be used outside of the exercise period as a snack. Plan a daily hydrating schedule of at least six 12 ounce glasses of water.

Section 9: Fighting and Overcoming Aging

Aging—a naturally degenerative disease—begins in adulthood and takes a quantum leap after the age of fifty. You can prevent and correct this disease to a great extent by taking antioxidant vitamins and herbs in addition to healthy foods and exercise.

Scientists after many years of research, can positively proclaim that antioxidants can dramatically reverse the inevitable consequences of aging—signs of physical deterioration and disease. For example, this research has shown amazing results in reducing:

homocystine (an amino acid in the blood)—the body produces more as we age and it causes blood clots, immunity deficiencies, the impact of thymus gland shrinking and age related brain dysfunctions.

The major cause of aging lies in the free radical theory. It virtually encompasses every disease connected with growing older. A free radical is a molecule that has lost one of its electrically charged electrons. In attempting to balance itself, the radical steals an electron from other molecules or allows an impaired electron to freely go off on its own. This event creates a molecular destructive chain reaction. Impacts on the DNA, especially in the mitochondria, can cause mutations that produce aberrant cell behavior. Over time, free radical mayhem takes its toll by leaving the body aged and diseased.

The knights in shining armor are antioxidants. The antioxidant donates a sorely-needed electron to a free radical without it becoming harmful. Putting this very simply, the antioxidant puts an end to the destructiveness of the free radical and puts the brakes on aging.

As we get older, it becomes more difficult to fight off free radicals. Two critical things happen biologically. The free radical rate of increase accelerates dramatically. At the same time, the basic abilities to defuse and repair free radical damage become less effective. Therefore, the need to bolster our free radical defenses actually becomes a life or death situation.

There are three ways to neutralize this free radical free-for-all.

First: Eat plenty of antioxidants so that you can flood the blood stream and then on to your cells with neutralizers of free radicals. Be sure to include the four powerful antioxidants—vitamin C, vitamin D, vitamin E and beta carotene as well as foods such as broccoli, tomatoes, tea and garlic. Recent studies have discovered that vitamin D is vital for health and longevity. Without sufficient amounts of this vitamin, you are more susceptible to the development of arterial plaque. This causes an increased risk of heart attacks and strokes.

Second: Avoid foods that are easily oxidized—they generate free radicals inside your cells and destroy them. These include corn and safflower oil, margarine and dried eggs found in many processed foods.

Third: Ingest herbs, vitamin supplements and other foods that directly stimulate enzymes to ramp up the body's detoxification systems which zap free radicals.

By feeding your cells antioxidants, you provide them a powerful "youth" elixir.

It is very important to note that a healthy diet can deliver great nutrition. However, achieving therapeutic levels of nutrients realistically will never happen without adding vitamin supplements and herbs to your diet. Seeking the advice from a nutritionist on what is best for you should get you on the right track in fighting aging and its impact.

In summary, think of aging and its consequences as partly a vitamin-herb "deficiency disease". The main way vitamins and herbs combat aging is by boosting antioxidant activity and crushing free radicals. The really good news is: vitamins and herbs in anti-aging doses are safe and free from side effects. Unless you follow some of the suggestions mentioned above, aging and disease will prevent you from running into your 90's and beyond.

My personal experience has shown that vitamin supplements and herbs are absolutely essential after you reach fifty-five years of age for your joints, eyes, energy and a healthy heart.

Section 10: Brain Aerobics and Nutrition

If you don't exercise the brain separately, you will lose its vital functions. It is very important to establish a daily mental calisthenics program.

This needs to involve a mental process that actively weighs and calculates different ideas or courses of action. Activities that you should consider are: crosswords and other word games, Sudoku, bridge—preferably duplicate bridge, chess and, believe it or not, surfing the web. In addition, physical exercise is very critical. In a 2008 Australian *JAMA* study it was found that when people with mild memory problems exercised 50 minutes three times a week, their cognitive function was enhanced. The exercise was only mildly aerobic—mostly just walking.

Exercise provides significant benefits. It improves blood flow to the brain which consumes about 20 percent of the oxygen and glucose you ingest. Physical activity also helps control blood pressure and weight. It helps in fighting diabetes. When diabetes occurs before age 65, this doubles the risk of Alzheimer's disease. Another concern is abdominal obesity during midlife which triples the risk of dementia at age 70.

One really good piece of positive news for older persons is that Scandinavian scientists recently discovered that drinking three to five cups of caffeinated coffee a day leads to a 65% reduction in the risk of developing dementia.

Another study in Britain showed that persons over 65 who tested with low levels of vitamin D were more than twice as likely to have increased cognitive problems.

Moreover, a good nutritional supplement program is essential to avoid poor memory problems. For example, vitamin B12 helps fight brain shrinkage and reduces the risk of dementia. Vitamin B3 lowers levels of protein connected with Alzheimer's. Folic acid and vitamins B6 and B12 keep toxic homocysteine in check. Several other supplements such as fish oil and curcumin also play a significant role. The bottom line is most Americans are at greater risk to Alzheimer's and dementia due to deficiencies in supplements and diet. Now is a good time to consult a good nutritionist and get yourselves in the low risk ballpark for these diseases.

Section 11: Experience

I started running on a regular basis when I was a Major in the US Army assigned to the Pentagon in 1971. I was put on orders to go to parachute training (jump school) in 1972. So in 1971 I began my preparatory training by running several miles a day in combat boots!!! I continued to run in the service until I retired in 1979. After that I discovered road races in Northern Virginia and have continued to participate in 5k, 8k, 10k and 15k races over the years.

I have overcome many injuries and physical problems after reaching the age of 55. At 55 years, *plantar fasciitis* came at me with a vengeance. I would wake up in the morning after a long run—10 to 12 miles in those days—with the bottom of my feet burning and in great pain. A trip to the podiatrist revealed that this ailment was due to my flat feet. Molded inserts were made and introduced to my running and walking shoes. This problem was completely taken care of. You should note that factors that predispose you to *plantar fasciitis* are tight calf muscles, tight hamstrings, prolonged running or walking on hard surfaces and over-pronation.

Then at the age of 57 my knees started to stiffen up and caused me to cut back on my running. At that time my son and my daughter talked me into doing mini-triathlons with them. This accidentally introduced me to cross training. Doing the cycling and swimming caused the stiffness in my knees to go away. I have included cross training in my weekly training regimen ever since.

At the age of 66 I had a torn rotator cuff in my right shoulder. Even though the pain was quite acute, I continued to run road races. I remember in 2001 trying to run the Sallie Mae 10k in Washington DC. After a ½ mile my hamstring muscles in my right leg were very painfully affected by this condition—so I stopped running. After the rotator cuff was repaired by surgery, I returned to active road racing without any problems. Then, at age 69, I developed osteo-arthritis in my right knee.

My orthopedic surgeon confirmed the condition with an MRI. Fortunately, my nutritionist's newsletter had an article which described an identical problem. It suggested taking 550 mgs. of ginger root every day as a solution. I began taking the ginger root in capsule form and in 5 weeks time, my arthritis was no longer a problem! I still continue to take ginger root on a daily basis. Later at 72, I developed a serious tightening and pain in the glutes, hamstrings and quadriceps on my right leg. My sports therapist resolved the situation after two visits. The problem was that my right leg, when running, was swinging out to the right due to weak inner thigh muscles. By introducing repetitions on the adduction exercise machine in my two weekly weight resistance workouts, I was able to correct the problem and return to a full running schedule. Lastly, at 73 my glutes on the right side started acting up again. This time my sports therapist discovered four muscles on the upper ham strings were counter tightening in response to my running workouts. He devised a special stretching procedure which I use prior to and after running which seems to loosen these muscles and not hamper the running exercise.

The moral of the above experiences is find a top notch sports therapist and your dreams of running until you are 100 years old may not be just a figment of your imagination!!!

Section 12: Summary of Major Factors That Will Contribute to Your Running Until 100 Years Old

After you reach 55 years of age, you should look at following a structured training/race schedule. Tailor your schedule that fits your needs and circumstances. You may want to consider including some or all of the following:

Restrict your hard workouts and runs to 60 minutes. Don't run back-to-back days. Take 1 to 2 days of rest each week. Include one cross training day in your weekly regimen. Schedule two weight resistance workouts in your weekly training. Your long training run should be a mile longer than your next racing distance but not more than 60 minutes.

Incorporate interval training into your schedule to reinforce the race pace.

Don't run on concrete surfaces. Make sure your running shoes have been properly evaluated and fitted. Consider getting a full complement of vitamin supplements and herbs to offset the debilitating effects of aging.

Visit a certified sports therapist every three to four months for "periodic maintenance" services. Take steps to insure that your memory is "sharp as a tack" and that your diet and supplements are geared to prevent dementia.

Remember—if you take care of your body, your body will take care of you.

Author's Note

Of significance is noting the recent federal government's Physical Activity Guidelines Advisory Committee findings on Functional Health, Mental Health and Bone Health. The panel recommended that major benefits for each category occur by including between 90 minutes and five hours per week of aerobic and strength training exercises.